Diabetic Meal Prep Cookbook For Beginners

Proven Strategies On Delicious Diabetic Recipes To Reverse Type 2 Diabetes, Boost Weight Loss And Ensure Total Body Healing With Simple And Healthy Diabetes Meals

Joanna Castillo

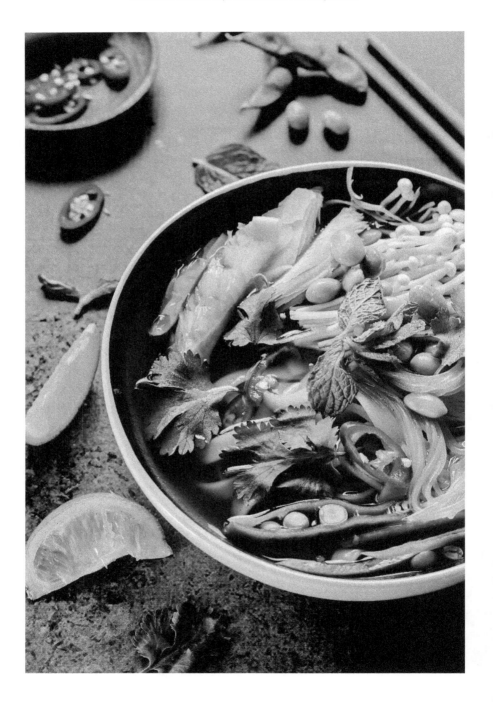

Contents

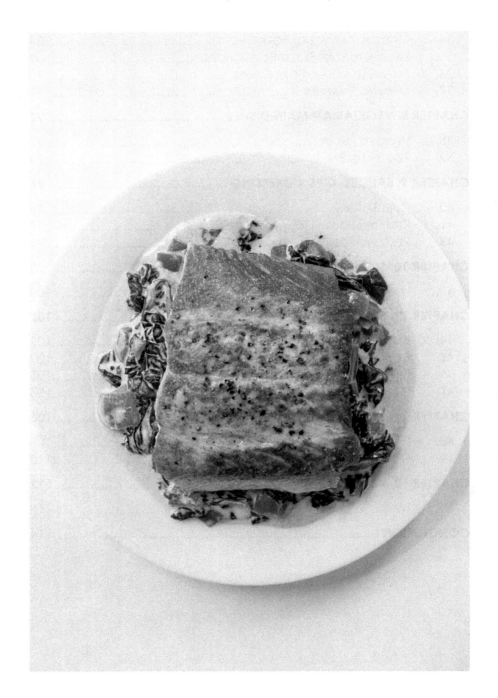

Introduction

Kudos for your achievement. You've made the first step toward overcoming diabetes, which is a life-threatening illness. Since diabetes is too common, we can no longer take a passive path to regain our well-being. This book is about those who want to take decisive steps in their fight to shed a significant amount of weight and cure diabetes, hypertension, and heart disease. You have the power to take control of your life. It's in your control. We will begin right now if we work together. Type 2 (adult-onset) diabetes may be prevented and recovered fully.

You probably have a procedure in place as a person with diabetes to stay on top of the condition with glucose control, routine medical appointments, and drug changes. These tried-and-true methods for maintaining blood glucose regulation are regarded as critical to your well-being. Unfortunately, this is completely incorrect. Instead of studying ways to get rid of diabetes, your life and these medications regulate your blood sugar. And if you have good glucose regulation, if you have diabetes, you can age prematurely and live a shorter existence. Furthermore, focusing solely on the numbers rather than addressing the root causes of diabetes can exacerbate the condition in the long run.

The bulk of blood-sugar-lowering drugs put a strain on your pancreas, which is still weakening. Since drugs used to regulate blood glucose levels, such as sulfonylureas and insulin, can induce weight gain, the likelihood of your diabetes worsening under traditional medical treatment is particularly high. As you get more diabetic, the risky combination of forcing the pancreas to generate insulin and still losing weight on drugs potentially leads to the need for more medication. This tried-and-true method reduces life expectancy and raises the likelihood of heart attacks.

In the United States, the percentage of individuals with diabetes (Type 2) has increased in the past thirty years. The primary cause for this is well-known: America's growing waistline. Despite this, doctors, dieticians, and even the American Medical Association (AMA) have all but abandoned weight reduction as a primary diabetes therapy. The drug remains the standard of care, including the fact that it is also the medication that causes weight gain, worsens effects, and makes people diabetic. This leads to a vicious cycle:

- As a person's diabetes progresses, more prescriptions are required.
- The doses increase.
- The person develops diabetes.

It's a blunder when it comes to our welfare. Most diabetic patients would've been safer off if these drugs had never been developed, so they would have been compelled to adjust their diet and dietary patterns as a result. On a personal and national basis, there is no need for a drug to reverse and avoid diabetes. It necessitates a change in our eating habits.

Since conventional diets don't succeed, the medical profession has given up on weight reduction to treat diabetics. Because, even though you've tried and struggled at a variety of diets in the past, don't give up.

The diet plan outlined on these pages is successful. You'll see a significant change in your fitness. Your body belongs to you, and you need it. With the lifesaving dietary material in this book, you will cure and even eradicate your diabetes.

We've been using the same dietary strategy for over ten thousand patients for over twenty years, and it's built on one core concept:

Nutrients (N) / Calories (C) = Your Health Future (H)

Our process is very different from some and has been shown to operate.

We'll show you how, if you offer your body the right resources, it will cure itself. The truth is that your body is designed for health. It transforms into a miraculous self-healing system when given the correct biochemical environment for healing.

Our method is founded on a mathematical algorithm for calculating life expectancy and fitness. This formula, defined as $H=N/C$, states that the nutrient-per-calorie amount of your food determines your fitness.

Your fitness will change significantly, and your diabetes will disappear if you consume more high-nutrient-density foods and less low-nutrient-density foods.

The body ages more slowly and is well equipped to avoid and reverse certain common ailments as you consume only high-nutrient diets. The innate self-healing and self-repairing power that has been dormant in your body awakens and gains over, and diseases vanish. The trick to maintaining optimum weight and fitness is to eat a nutrient-dense diet that includes green vegetables, tomatoes, beans, mushrooms, onions, nuts, and other natural foods.

Contrary to public belief, the numerous illnesses that afflict all and endanger our lives are not a natural part of aging. We aren't the product of bad breeding. We don't need a constant supply of pills during our lives.

We've come to assume that our disease-causing excess body fat is natural, appropriate, and impossible to lose. Drugs aren't the answer to weight gain, asthma, or other issues that tend to accompany aging.

Control comes from knowledge. You will get healthier, live much longer, and sleep happier every day by understanding how you consume impact your fitness and well-being. The effects of my software astound all who use it.

CHAPTER 1: Diabetic Diet Overview

Our fitness, strength, and well-being are all influenced by what we eat. Glucose is formed after various carbohydrates are broken down and absorbed into the bloodstream. The pancreas releases insulin to keep our blood glucose levels from being too elevated or too low. If you are suffering from diabetes (Type 2), the pancreas isn't producing sufficient insulin, or the insulin you have isn't working properly.

Diet is good for everyone, but it is especially important for people with Type 2 diabetes. Choosing the right foods will help you control your diabetes and reduce the chances of developing other health conditions.

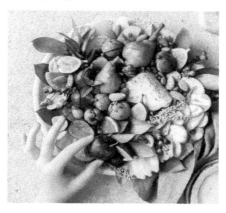

According to one report, people with Diabetes (Type 2) could lower their blood glucose levels by an average of 25% by adopting a simple diet plan close to the one we prescribe. While healthier and harmful foods are often discussed, there is no such thing as good or poor food;

what matters is the balance of foods consumed during the day.

1. Diabetes Type 2 (T2D):

Type 2 diabetes, formerly known as adult-onset diabetes, started at the age of 40, although it is now more common in teenagers, who are more overweight and exercise less. The trouble with diabetes (Type 2) isn't a complete deficiency of insulin-like it is with type 1, but more insulin resistance, which means the glucose doesn't get into the cells and stays in the blood.

2. What Is the Glycemic Index (GI), Precisely?

The glycemic index (GI) is related to the number of carbohydrates throughout a meal. But it's not so much a test of carbohydrate quantities as it is of carbohydrate efficiency. It is a specific indicator of how carbohydrates in foods influence blood glucose levels. When we use the word blood sugar, like I did a few paragraphs before, we are just talking about glucose.

That's the most basic kind of sugar, and the accumulation of it in the blood is what we're talking about when we say "blood sugar amounts."

Other more complex sugars and starches, or carbohydrates, are converted to glucose to use the body by the digestive method.

The glycemic index determines how fast the mechanism occurs with various foods. High-GI foods break down rapidly, allowing blood glucose levels to rise. Lower-GI diets digest more steadily but over a prolonged period, causing blood glucose levels to fluctuate less.

In general, select items with a lower glycemic index to keep blood glucose levels as stable as possible. Whole-grain bread, unrefined cereals (such as oats), and basmati rice are examples of carbohydrate sources of lower glycemic indexes. The Glycemic index is even smaller in cookies, cakes, and muffins made from fruits and whole grains.

It's almost difficult to predict a blended meal's glycemic index (one that includes an appetizer, a main course, and a dessert). Still, you might lower the diet's glycemic index with a few easy substitutions.

3. Why Is GI Important?

Consuming more low-GI diets is a smart thing for most individuals. If an individual has diabetes or some glucose resistance, they may not have the same blood glucose spikes. As a result of these surges, the body produces more insulin than is needed.

After the high-GI diet has had little effect on blood glucose levels, the insulin level stays high. Lower-GI diets allow glucose and insulin levels to fluctuate less during the day, putting fewer burdens on the body. And is often beneficial to one's cardiac well-being.

High insulin levels have been related to elevated blood pressure and cholesterol levels in studies. High glucose levels can cause cells to become stressed, resulting in inflammatory responses that may lead to blood clots and artery blockages.

4. Diabetic Diet Advantages

To recap, below are some of the main health advantages of a diabetic diet:

- **Assist with Controlling Diabetes**

Diabetes is a disease that affects people. This is one of the first advantages we see while considering a low-GI diet. Choosing foods that are digested more slowly reduces blood glucose fluctuations and the subsequent insulin spikes. As you eliminate the roller-coaster influence, the body is less anxious, and you sleep healthier, and your glucose and insulin levels are more stable. Furthermore, low-GI diets provide fewer sugars total, which is beneficial to those suffering from glucose sensitivity.

- **Weight Loss**

This topic has recently sparked a lot of attention. A variety of diets have concentrated on lowering carbohydrate intake. When we speak of low-GI diets, it is not what we prescribe.

We're going to focus on the carbohydrates you consume. While a low-GI diet can have fewer total carbohydrates, the main advantage is the slower digestion of low-GI foods. This ensures you're less likely to get hungry again right after feeding and want another high-GI fix to feel complete and happy.

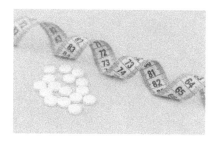

- **Cardiovascular Health**

A low-GI diet often has a host of heart-healthy effects, some of which are overt and indirect. First and foremost, many of the foods we'll discuss on a low-GI diet are the same ones I discussed in my 500 Reduced Recipes book. Low-GI foods include whole grains, legumes, fruits, and vegetables, which can help reduce cholesterol levels.

A high insulin level, such as those produced by a high-GI diet, may also lead to higher cholesterol levels and promotes the deposit of fatty acids in the arteries, increasing the risk of stroke and heart attack, as previously reported. A low-GI diet can assist with various risk factors for heart disease, including cholesterol levels, diabetes or prediabetes, and becoming overweight.

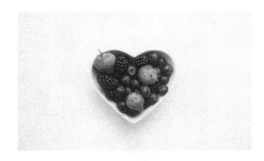

5. Foods to Eat and to Stay Away From

Let's get down to the nitty-gritty of what foods you can consume and what foods you should skip keeping the average glycemic index low.

Let's start with some basic descriptions of some items' glycemic index and then move on to some general characteristics that appear to make a product have a lower or higher GI.

Some Low-GI Foods (GI less than 55) and Their Respective Glycemic Index

- Yogurt, low fat (sweetened) 14
- Zucchini 15
- Celery 15
- Cauliflower 15
- Broccoli 15
- Asparagus 15
- Artichoke 15
- Cherries 22
- Grapefruit 25

- Pearl barley 25
- Chickpeas 33
- Milk, skim 32
- Apricots (dried) 31
- Soy milk 30
- Kidney beans boiled 29
- Milk, whole 27
- Oranges 44
- Peaches 42
- All-Bran 42
- Plums 39
- Wheat kernels 41
- Apple juice 41
- Black-eyed beans 41
- Carrots cooked 39
- Pears 38
- Apples 38
- Spaghetti, whole wheat 37
- Spinach 15
- Rice, instant 46
- Peppers, all varieties 15
- Grapefruit juice 48
- Green beans 15

- Whole grain 50
- Cucumber 15
- Yam 51
- Bananas 54
- Kiwifruit 53
- Sweet potato 54
- Orange juice 52
- Eggplant 15
- Barley cracked 50
- Lettuce, all varieties 15
- Multigrain bread 48
- Spaghetti, durum wheat 55
- Rice, brown 55
- Grapes 46
- Oat bran 55
- Tomatoes 15
- Macaroni 45
- Fruit cocktail 55
- Snow peas 15

Some Medium-GI Foods (GI between 56 and 69) and Their Respective Glycemic Index

- Muffin (unsweetened) 62
- Mangoes 56

- Pizza, cheese 60
- Pita bread, white 57
- Rice, white 58
- Potato, new 57
- Apricots 57
- Danish pastry 59
- Rice, wild 57
- Hamburger bun 61
- Potato boiled 56
- Rye-flour bread 64
- Muesli 56

Some High-GI Foods (GI 70 and Above) and Their Respective Glycemic Index

- Baguette 95
- Golden Grahams 71
- Cornflakes 83
- Potato chips 75
- Rice Kris pies 82
- Doughnut 76
- Waffles 76
- Potato baked 85
- Puffed Wheat 74
- Parsnips 97

- White bread 71

We will begin to draw certain generalizations on the types of foods we should and should not consume by looking down this page. Let's have a peek at a few groups and some suggestions for each.

Fruits and vegetables

Fruits and vegetables, with a few variations, are excellent low-GI foods. A few bananas, such as pineapple and apricots, have a medium to large GI, as do potatoes, but nearly all other foods have a low GI.

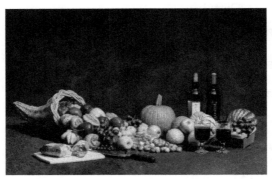

Legume

Low-GI legumes include kidney beans, chickpeas, lentils, and a variety of other legumes. They're excellent options because the fiber content tends to slow digestion and prevent you from being hungry over prolonged periods. They often provide high-quality, fat-free protein, which means they cram a ton of nutrients into a small number of calories.

Baked Goods and Grains

We've arrived at a point where being picky pays off. White flour and refined grain brands have a much higher GI than whole-grain alternatives. This is due to two factors. First, heavily modified grains also had a considerable amount of fiber eliminated, resulting in a higher GI ranking and better digestion.

Second, they're typically pounded into even smaller pieces. This also allows them easy to eat, which means their carbs are processed into glucose faster, raising the GI number and making you hungry quicker.

This is true not only of white bread but also of the more refined breakfast cereals.

Sweets

There aren't many of these on the chart, but they're areas where you can be extra cautious. They have a higher GI, which gives you a fast yet fleeting boost. They often happen to be low in nutrients, producing empty calories that contribute to weight gain but not good health. I've added several recipes for low-GI treats that you can enjoy in moderation, but if you want anything tasty, go for an apple or a pot of yogurt instead of a candy bar.

6. Hypertension

Hypertension is a condition under which the blood pressure increases in the arteries. Arteries are blood vessels that transport blood from the beating heart to all your body's tissues and organs. While emotional tension and stress may momentarily raise blood pressure, high blood pressure does not often equal serious mental tension.

7. **Hypertension Natural Treatments:**

High blood pressure, if left unchecked, increases the chances of heart failure and stroke. And without drugs, there are many steps you may do to naturally lower the blood pressure. Here are several traditional means for lowering blood pressure.

Stop Smoking:

Smoking is a major risk factor for heart failure and is one of the causes to stop. A breath of tobacco smoke raises blood pressure for a brief period. Tobacco chemicals have also been linked to blood vessel injury.

Surprisingly, there hasn't been a definitive correlation between smoking and high blood pressure in the research. This may be how smokers build up resistance over time. Smoking and high blood pressure also increase the likelihood of heart failure, so avoiding smoking will help reduce the risk.

Lose Weight:

For overweight individuals, losing weight will make a significant improvement in their cardiac wellbeing. A 2016 research found that reducing 5% of the bodyweight would dramatically reduce high blood pressure. Previous research has connected losing 17.64 pounds (8 kilograms) to lower systolic and diastolic blood pressure by 8.5 and 6.5 mm Hg, respectively.

A safe reading should be less than 120/80 mm Hg to bring that into context. When weight reduction is combined with exercise, the result is much stronger. Losing weight will make the blood vessels widen and compress more easily, making it simpler for the left ventricle of your heart to pump blood.

Consume Dark Chocolate:

Dark chocolate is high in flavanols, which relax blood vessels and increase blood flow, and evidence indicates that eating dark chocolate regularly may help lower blood pressure. According to Mo, chocolate shouldn't be the primary method for controlling blood pressure, but it is a safe option when you need a treat.

Stress Management:

High blood pressure is exacerbated by stress. When you're nervous all the time, your body is always in fight-or-flight mode. Physically, this translates to a higher heart rhythm and constricted blood vessels. Because you're stressed, you're more inclined to indulge in risky habits like consuming too much alcohol or eating unhealthy foods that can raise your blood pressure.

Reduce Caffeine:

Whether you've just enjoyed a cup of coffee since having your blood pressure taken, you'll realize the caffeine gives you a lift right away. However, there isn't much proof that consuming caffeine daily will lead to a long-term boost.

On the other hand, caffeine and coffee drinkers have a smaller chance of heart failure, like elevated blood pressure, than non-drinkers. Caffeine can have a greater impact on individuals who do not routinely drink it.

Reduce the Alcohol Consumption:

Alcohol consumption will increase blood pressure. In reality, alcohol is related to 16% of all cases of high blood pressure worldwide. Although some evidence suggests that low-to-moderate alcohol levels can be beneficial to the heart, the advantages can be outweighed by negative consequences.

Eat Foods High in Potassium:

Potassium is a vital element. It aids in the removal of sodium from the body and relieves blood flow pressure. Many people's sodium consumption has improved, although their potassium intake has decreased due to modern diets. Focus on consuming less refined foods and more new, whole foods to achieve a healthier potassium-to-sodium ratio in your diet. Beans, vegetables, particularly potatoes, tomatoes, leafy greens, and sweet potatoes, for example, are high in potassium. Fruit, such as bananas, melons, tomatoes, avocados, and apricots dairies, such as yogurt and milk seeds and nuts

Reduce the Salt Intake:

In the globe, people consume a lot of salt. Processed and prepared goods are to blame for a substantial part of this. As a result, several public policy initiatives are targeted at reducing salt consumption in the food sector. High salt consumption has been related in several researches to high blood pressure and cardiac events, including stroke.

However, a recent study suggests that the connection between sodium and high blood pressure is less obvious. One cause for this may be hereditary variations in sodium metabolism. Salt exposure seems to affect half of the people with elevated blood pressure and a fifth of people with low blood pressure.

Enjoy walking and workout:

Exercise is one of the most effective ways to reduce elevated blood pressure. Regular activity strengthens and improves the heart pumps' efficiency, lowering blood pressure in the arteries. In reality, 150 minutes a week of moderate exercise, such as walking, or 75 minutes per week of intense exercises, such as running, will help reduce blood pressure and boost heart health.

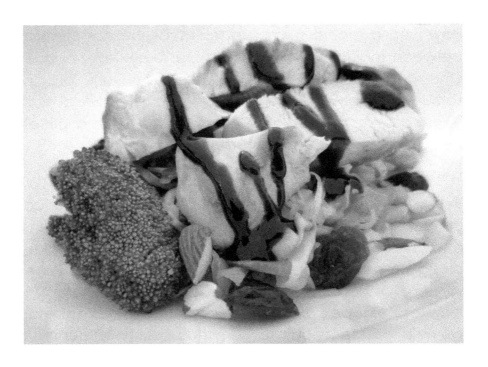

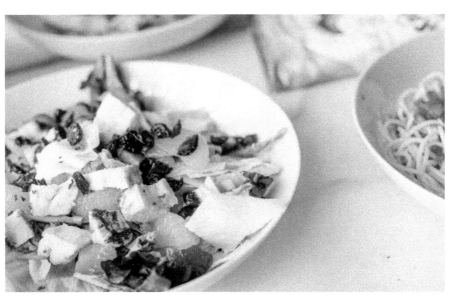

CHAPTER 2: The 21-Day Meal Plan

Day 1

Breakfast

- Soaked Oats and Blueberries

Lunch

- Fresh fruit (strawberries)
- Yum Good Beans
- Tofu Ranch Dressing/Dip
- Salad with mixed greens and veggies

Dinner

- Fresh fruit (apple slices with cinnamon)
- Herbed Barley and Lentils
- The Big Veggie Stir-Fry

Day 2

Breakfast

- Blue Apple Nut Oatmeal

Lunch

- Fresh fruit (Grapes)
- French Lentil Soup
- Mixed greens salad with assorted vegetables and flavored vinegar

Dinner

- Mango Coconut Sorbet
- French Lentil Soup
- Herbed White Bean Hummus
- Raw veggies

Day 3

Breakfast

- Quick Banana Oat Breakfast to Go

Lunch

- Fresh fruit (apple slices and cinnamon)
- Anticancer Soup
- Island Black Bean Dip
- Raw vegetables

Dinner

- Fresh fruit or Banana Walnut Ice Cream
- Anticancer Soup
- Island Black Bean Dip
- Raw vegetables

Day 4

Breakfast

- Fruit and nut bowl (assorted fresh and frozen fruit topped with nuts or seeds)

Lunch

- Fresh fruit (grapes)
- Savory Portobello Mushrooms with Chickpeas
- Mixed greens salad with assorted vegetables and flavored vinegar

Dinner

- Fresh fruit (berries)
- Eggplant Roll-Ups
- Tofu Ranch Dressing/Dip
- Romaine, spinach, and watercress salad

Day 5

Breakfast

- Walnuts
- Blended Mango Salad

Lunch

- Fresh fruit (two kiwis)
- Black Bean Lettuce Bundles
- Russian Fig Dressing/Dip
- Raw vegetables

Dinner

- Mixed berries
- Roasted Vegetable Salad with Baked Tofu or Salmon
- Seasoned edamame

Day 6

Breakfast

- Fruit and nut bowl (assorted fresh and frozen fruit topped with nuts and seeds)

Lunch

- Fresh fruit (orange)
- Golden Austrian Cauliflower Cream Soup
- Russian Fig Dressing/Dip
- Romaine, spinach, and watercress salad topped with chickpeas

Dinner

- Peach Sorbet
- Great Greens
- Simple Bean Burgers
- Fresh Tomato Salsa
- Raw vegetables

Day 7

Breakfast

- Soaked Oats and Blueberries

Lunch

- Fresh fruit (apple)
- Salad with romaine lettuce, mixed greens, and assorted vegetables topped with white beans Caesar Salad Dressing/Dip

Dinner

- Fresh fruit (melon)
- Golden Austrian Cauliflower Cream Soup
- Steamed asparagus with Sesame Ginger Sauce

Day 8

Breakfast

- Blue Apple Nut Oatmeal

Lunch

- Fresh fruit (blueberries)
- Easy Bean and Vegetable Chili
- Romaine and mixed greens salad and flavored vinegar

Dinner

- Fresh fruit (cherries)
- Choice of cooked vegetable with Almond Tomato Sauce*

- Mushroom Soup Provencal

Day 9

Breakfast

- Fruit and nut bowl

Lunch

- Fresh fruit (pear)
- Vegetable Burrito
- Creamy Blueberry Dressing
- Romaine and arugula salad with assorted vegetables

Dinner

- Easy Bean and Vegetable Chili
- Choice of healthy dips
- Strawberries dusted with cocoa powder
- Raw vegetables

Day 10

Breakfast

- Blue Apple Nut Oatmeal

Lunch

- Speedy Vegetable Wrap
- Thousand Island Dressing
- Romaine, spinach, and watercress salad

Dinner

- Braised Baby Bok Choy
- Pistachio-Crusted Tempeh with Balsamic Marinade and Shiitake Mushrooms
- Fresh Tomato Salsa
- Blueberry Cobbler
- Raw vegetables

Day 11

Breakfast

- Green Gorilla Blended Salad

Lunch

- Fresh fruit (watermelon slices)
- Mushroom Soup Provencal
- Choice of healthy dips
- Raw vegetables

Dinner

- Mediterranean Bean and Kale Sauté
- Green Velvet Dressing/Dip
- Steamed artichoke

Day 12

Breakfast

- Fruit and nut bowl

Lunch

- Fresh fruit (orange)
- Asparagus Polonaise
- Fast Mexican Black Bean Soup

Dinner

- Garlicky Zucchini
- Caesar Salad Dressing/Dip
- Low-sodium marinara sauce

- No-Meat Balls
- Fresh fruit (pear)
- Romaine salad with assorted vegetables

Day 13

Breakfast

- Nut or seed topping
- Tropical Fruit Salad

Lunch

- Fresh fruit (apple)
- Southern-Style Mixed Greens

Dinner

8. Fresh fruit (melon)
9. Swiss Chard with Garlic and Lemon
10. Fast Mexican Black Bean Soup

Day 14

Breakfast

- Quick Banana Oat Breakfast to Go

Lunch

- Fresh fruit (papaya)
- Steamed vegetable of choice with Red Lentil Sauce
- Flavored vinegar or choice of healthy dressings
- Mixed greens salad

Dinner

- Strawberry Pineapple Sorbet
- Thai Vegetable Curry
- Choice of healthy dips
- Raw vegetables

Day 15

Breakfast

- Apple Kale Smoothie
- Zucchini Pancakes

Lunch

- Fresh fruit (melon)
- Roasted Beet Salad
- Lemon Pork with Asparagus
- Mixed greens salad

Dinner

- Garlicky Zucchini
- Caesar Salad Dressing/Dip
- Low-sodium marinara sauce
- No-Meat Balls
- Fresh fruit (pear)
- Romaine salad with assorted vegetables

Day 16

Breakfast

- Flax Almond Butter Smoothie
- Naan Pancakes Crepes

Lunch

- Fresh fruit (grapes)
- Pomegranate Avocado salad
- Easy Lentil Dhal

Dinner

11. Fresh fruit (melon)
12. Kale Pork
13. Egg-Drop Soup

Day 17

Breakfast

14. Cacao Spinach Smoothie
15. Egg Bake

Lunch

- Fresh fruit (melon)
- Mediterranean Salad
- Vegetarian Chili

Dinner

16. Fresh fruit (kiwi)
17. White Chicken Chili

18. Avgolemono – Greek lemon chicken soup

Day 18

Breakfast

19. Broccoli Leeks Cucumber smoothie

20. Smoked Salmon Scrambled Eggs

Lunch

- Fresh fruit (strawberries)
- Greek Cucumber Salad
- Spinach Rolls

Dinner

21. Fresh fruit (apple)

22. Turkey Sausage and Pepper Patties

23. Kale White Bean Pork Soup

Day 19

Breakfast

- Beet Greens Smoothie
- Omelet with veggies

Lunch

- Fresh fruit (banana)
- Cauliflower & Eggs Salad
- Cheese Pie

Dinner

24. Fresh fruit (berry)
25. Turkey Meat Loaf
26. Squash Soup

Day 20

Breakfast

- Watercress Smoothie
- Egg pizza crust

Lunch

- Fresh fruit (orange)
- Quinoa Salad
- Mushroom and Pepper Quiche

Dinner

27. Fresh fruit (melon)
28. White Bean and Smoked Turkey Casserole

29. Black Bean Soup

Day 21

Breakfast

- Avocado Kale Smoothie
- Coconut Pomegranate Oatmeal

Lunch

- Fresh fruit (banana)
- Southern-Style Mixed Greens
- Beef Stew with Peas and Carrots

Dinner

30. Fresh fruit (kiwi)

31. Spanish Chicken Thighs

32. Creamy Roasted Mushroom

CHAPTER 3: Breakfast & Brunch Recipes

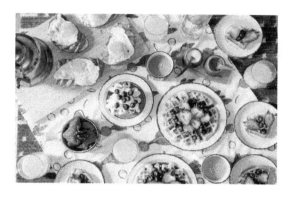

1. Cranberry Apricot Waffles

Preparation time: 10 minutes

Cooking time: 10 minutes

Servings: 2 servings

Ingredients:

- 1 cup cranberry juice
- 1/2 teaspoon baking powder
- 3 tablespoons sugar
- 1 cup cottage cheese
- 16 ounces apricot halves
- 4 egg whites, stiffly beaten
- 1 tablespoon unsalted butter, melted
- 2 tablespoons cornstarch

- 4 egg yolks
- 1/4 teaspoon almond extract
- 1/2 cup flour

Directions:

1. Combine flour and baking powder in a sifter. Combine the next three products, as well as the flour mixture, in a mixer. Blend until fully smooth.

2. Fold the egg whites into the batter. Bake in a waffle maker that has been preheated. Apricots can be drained and chopped up, with the juice saved.

3. Combine sugar and cornstarch in a saucepan. Mix with the apricot and cranberry juices. Cook, often stirring, until the sauce is rich and bubbly. Combine the extract and apricots in a mixing bowl. Heat the sauce and spill it over the waffles.

2. Cornmeal Pancakes

Preparation time: 10 minutes

Cooking time: 10 minutes

Servings: 7 servings

Ingredients:

- 1/4 teaspoon baking soda
- 3/4 cup cornmeal
- 1 tablespoon baking powder
- 1 cup whole wheat pastry flour
- 2 eggs
- 1 and 1/4 cups buttermilk
- 1/4 cup canola oil
- 1 cup boiling water

Directions:

1. Pour the water over the cornmeal and swirl until it becomes thick. In a separate bowl, whisk together the buttermilk and eggs. Combine rice, baking powder, and baking soda in a mixing dish. Toss in with the cornmeal blend. Include the canola oil and mix well on a hot grill, fry.

3. Cottage Cheese Pancakes

Preparation time: 10 minutes

Cooking time: 10 minutes

Servings: 4 servings

Ingredients:

- 2 tablespoons butter, melted
- 3 eggs
- 1/4 cup skim milk
- 1 cup cottage cheese
- 1/4 teaspoon salt
- 1 cup flour
- 1/4 cup Splenda

Directions:

1. Combine the eggs, Splenda, and salt in a mixing bowl. Mix in the cottage cheese and cream thoroughly. Gradually apply the flour and continue to beat until the mixture is smooth.

2. Apply the melted butter and blend properly. Spoon spoonfuls of batter onto an oiled griddle. When finely browned, on the one hand, flip and brown on the other.

4. Veggie Frittata

Preparation time: 10 minutes

Cooking time: 12 minutes

Servings: 4 servings

Ingredients:

- 1/4 teaspoon black pepper
- 1/2 cup chopped onion
- 6 eggs 1 cup sliced zucchini
- 8 ounces sliced mushrooms
- 1 tablespoon parsley
- 1 cup broccoli florets
- 2 ounces Swiss cheese, shredded
- 1/2 cup chopped red bell pepper

Directions:

1. Using nonstick vegetable oil paint, coat a big ovenproof skillet. Stir-fry the broccoli, bell pepper, and onion until crisp-tender. Stir in the mushrooms and zucchini for another 1 to 2 minutes. Combine the eggs, parsley, and black pepper in a mixing bowl and spill over the vegetable mixture, spreading to cover fully.

2. Cook, covered, for 10 to 12 minutes over medium heat, or until eggs are almost set. Cheese can be sprinkled on top. Broil the skillet until the eggs are fixed, and the cheese is melted.

5. Cinnamon Apple Omelet

Preparation time: 10 minutes

Cooking time: 15 minutes

Servings: 2 servings

Ingredients:

- 1 tablespoon sour cream
- 3 eggs
- 1 tablespoon brown sugar
- 1/2 teaspoon cinnamon
- 1 tablespoon cream
- 1 apple, peeled and sliced thin
- 1 tablespoon unsalted butter, divided

Directions:

1. In a pan, melt 2 teaspoons sugar. Combine the apple, cinnamon, and brown sugar in a mixing bowl. Cook until the vegetables are soft.

2. Remove from the flame. Whip the eggs and cream together until light and fluffy; set aside. Make sure the pan is clean.

3. Melt the remaining butter and whisk in the egg mixture. Cook as though you were making an omelet. Switch the eggs until they are about to be flipped. Cover the middle of the eggs with sour cream, and finish with the apple mixture. Place the omelet on a plate and fold it over.

6. **Hash Brown Omelet**

Preparation time: 10 minutes

Cooking time: 15 minutes

Servings: 6 servings

Ingredients:

- 1 cup cheddar, shredded
- 1/4 cup skim milk
- 4 eggs
- 1/4 cup green pepper, chopped
- 1/4 cup onion, chopped
- 2 cups frozen hash brown potatoes
- 1/4 teaspoon pepper
- 4 slices bacon

Directions:

1. Cook bacon until crisp in a 10 or 12-inch skillet. Remove the bacon and leave any drippings. Brown the potatoes, onion, and green pepper in a skillet and press them into the pan's rim.

2. Pour the eggs, milk, and pepper over the potatoes. Cover with cheese and bacon crumbles. Cook over low heat, covered, until the egg is formed.

7. Italian Breakfast Casserole

Preparation time: 10 minutes

Cooking time: 35 minutes

Servings: 8 servings

Ingredients:

- 1/2 teaspoon oregano, crumbled
- 1 tablespoon butter
- 1 cup tomatoes, peeled and chopped
- 1 cup red onion, chopped
- 1 cup milk 8 ounces mozzarella cheese, shredded
- 12 eggs, beaten
- 1/2 teaspoon freshly ground pepper
- 4 ounces mushrooms, sliced
- 1-pound Italian sausage, casings removed

Directions:

1. Cook crumbled sausage in a skillet until it is no longer pink. Drain the water and set it aside in a pot. In a skillet, sauté the onion and mushrooms until soft but not orange.

2. Toss with the bacon.

3. Add together the remaining components thoroughly. Bake for 30 to 35 minutes, or until knife inserted in the middle comes out clean, in an oiled 9 x 13-inch pan at 400°F (200°C, or gas mark 6) pan.

CHAPTER 4: Snack Sweets, Desserts, and Drink Recipes

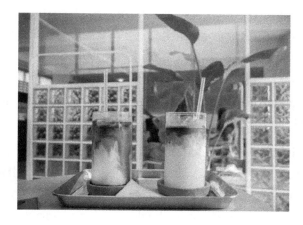

8. Peanut Butter Cookies

Preparation time: 10 minutes

Cooking time: 8-10 minutes

Servings: 18 serving

Ingredients:

- 1/2 cup sugar substitute, such as Splenda
- 1/4 teaspoon baking soda
- 4 tablespoons peanut butter
- 1/4 cup unsalted butter
- 1 tablespoon brown sugar substitute, such as Splenda
- 1/4 teaspoon baking powder
- 1 egg, well beaten

- 1/3 cup flour

Directions:

1. Preheat the oven to 375 degrees Fahrenheit (190 degrees Celsius, or gas mark 5). Lightly oil a baking sheet. Combine rice, baking soda, and baking powder in a sifter. With a whisk, combine the butter and peanut butter until creamy; progressively apply the brown sugar substitute, and function until light.

2. Mix in the granulated sugar substitute and the egg thoroughly. In a large mixing bowl, thoroughly combine the dry ingredients. Drop through teaspoonfuls onto a baking sheet and flatten in a criss-cross fashion with fork tines. Bake for 8-10 minutes or until completed.

9. Frozen Cherry Dessert

Preparation time: 10 minutes

Cooking time: 1 hour 10 minutes

Servings: 12 serving

Ingredients:

- 8 ounces plain fat-free yogurt
- 1 cup water, boiling
- 1 small box sugar-free gelatin, cherry flavor
- 2 cups whipped topping, like Cool Whip
- 8 ounces sweet cherries, undrained, pitted

Directions:

1. Plastic seal the bottom and sides of a 9 x 5-inch loaf pan and put it aside. Drain the cherries and set aside the sugar. Add sufficiently cool water to the reserved syrup to make 1/2 cup if required. Remove the pits from the cherries and break them into pieces.

2. In a pot of hot water, entirely remove gelatin. Pour in the sugar according to the measurements. Stir in the yogurt until it is thoroughly combined.

3. Chill for 45 minutes to an hour, stirring regularly, until the mixture has thickened but not hardened. Stir in the cherries and whipped topping gently.

4. Cover and pour into the prepared pot. Freeze for 6 hours or overnight before strong. 15 minutes before serving, take the tray out of the fridge.

Allow softening slightly at room temperature. Take off the bubble wrap.

5. Round the cake into slices. Leftovers can be covered and stored in the fridge.

CHAPTER 5: Salads & Appetizer Recipes

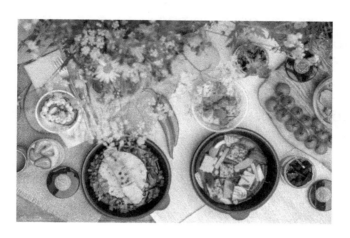

10. Hummus

Preparation time: 10 minutes

Cooking time: none

Servings: 8 servings

Ingredients:

- 1 tablespoon olive oil

- 1/2 teaspoon paprika

- 1 teaspoon cumin

- 1/4 cup tahini

- 1/4 cup water

- 3 tablespoons lemon juice

- 3 cloves garlic

- 1 cup cooked chickpeas

Directions:

1. In a food processor, combine the cooked chickpeas, garlic, lemon juice, and water. Blend for about a minute or until absolutely smooth. Add more water if it's too thick.

2. Taste and change the amount of lemon juice, tahini, cumin, and paprika as required. Drizzle olive oil over the top and spread it into a shallow dish. Chill before serving.

11. Green Onion Dip

Preparation time: 10 minutes

Cooking time: none

Servings: 8 servings

Ingredients:

- 2 teaspoons lemon juice
- 1/4 cup chopped green onion
- 1 cup cottage cheese

Directions:

In a blender or food processor, combine all of the ingredients and heat until smooth. Refrigerate for at least an hour before serving to encourage the flavors to meld.

12. Chile Con Queso

Preparation time: 10 minutes

Cooking time: 5 minutes

Servings: 12 servings

Ingredients:

- 2 teaspoons cumin, ground
- 2 tablespoons onion, finely chopped
- 1/4 cup half-and-half
- 4 ounces green chilies, chopped
- 1 cup cheddar cheese, shredded

Directions:

1. Heat all of the ingredients in a small saucepan over low heat, stirring continuously, until the cheese is fully melted. Serve with tortilla chips or vegetables when still warm.

13.   Apple Pecan Log

Preparation time: 10 minutes

Cooking time: none

Servings: 8 servings

Ingredients:

- 1 cup pecans, chopped
- 1 cup apple, chopped
- 1 teaspoon fresh lemon juice
- 1/2 teaspoon ground nutmeg
- 1 tablespoon apple juice
- 8 ounces cream cheese, softened

Directions:

1. In a mixer cup, combine cream cheese, apple juice, and nutmeg and beat until smooth. Add the chopped apples to the creamed cheese mixture after adding the lemon juice.

2. Fold in a cup of pecans gently, then roll into a 6-inch log and roll in the remaining chopped nuts. Wrap it in plastic wrap and keep it in the fridge until ready to serve.

14. Chicken Liver Pate

Preparation time: 10 minutes

Cooking time: 15 minutes

Servings: 10 servings

Ingredients:

- 2 ounces milk
- 1/8 teaspoon nutmeg
- 2 ounces sherry
- 4 tablespoons fresh rosemary
- 10 ounces chicken livers
- 1 clove minced garlic
- 1/2 cup finely chopped onion
- 4 slices low-sodium bacon
- 4 tablespoons olive oil

Directions:

1. In a large sauté pan, combine olive oil, bacon, and onion. On low heat, cook for 4 minutes before adding the garlic and liver. Cook for 15 minutes on medium heat. Allow 15 minutes for the rosemary and sherry to infuse or until the liver is completely cooked.

2. Allow cooling with a pinch of salt and nutmeg. Blend until smooth in a food processor. Stir in the milk slowly and pulse until smooth. On crostini, spread the jam.

15.   Roasted Red Pepper Spread

Preparation time: 10 minutes

Cooking time: 10 minutes

Servings: 6 servings

Ingredients:

- 2 tablespoons olive oil
- 1 garlic clove
- 12 ounces roasted red peppers, drained
- 1 slice whole-wheat bread, crusts trimmed

Directions:

1. Set aside bread that has been crumbled in a covered food processor container. Fill the container halfway with red peppers and garlic. Cover with plastic wrap and process until the mixture is completely smooth. Gradually add oil through the feed pote while the processor is running.

2. Cover and process until smooth with the reserved bread crumbs. Fill a small bowl with the mixture. With crackers or toasted bread, serve chilled or at room temperature.

16. Curried Cheese Spread

Preparation time: 10 minutes

Cooking time: 10 minutes

Servings: 10 servings

Ingredients:

- 1 tablespoon sherry
- 1 teaspoon curry powder
- 2 tablespoons tomato chutney
- 1 cup cheddar cheese, shredded
- 6 ounces cream cheese
- 1 tablespoon olive oil
- 1/4 cup onions, chopped

Directions:

1. In a skillet, soften onions in oil. Combine all of the ingredients in a large mixing bowl and chill until ready to use.

CHAPTER 6: Soup Recipes

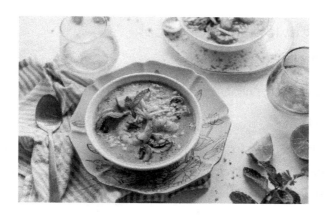

17.   Fish Chowder

Preparation time: 10 minutes

Cooking time: 30 minutes

Servings: 8 serving

Ingredients:

- 3 tablespoons unsalted butter, softened
- 1 pound perch
- 1 teaspoon parsley
- 1 onion, chopped
- 2 potatoes, cubed (optional)
- 1 clove garlic, minced
- 1 and 1/2 cups water
- 1 and 1/2 cups white wine
- 1/4 teaspoon thyme

- 1/2 cup chopped celery
- 3 tablespoons flour
- 4 slices low-sodium bacon
- 1/2 cup skim milk
- 1 pound salmon

Directions:

1. If the fish is frozen, thaw it and cube it. In a Dutch oven, cook bacon. Crumble the bread and put it aside. Remove most of the oil from the pot. Cook until the cabbage, celery, and garlic are soft. Combine the wine, sugar, potatoes (if using), and spices in a large mixing bowl.

2. Simmer for about 20 minutes, or until potatoes are almost finished. Add the tuna, cover, and cook for another 10 minutes. To make a paste, combine flour and butter. Stir into the broth and cook until it has thickened. In a separate bowl, combine the milk and the bacon that has been set aside.

18.   Fish Stew

Preparation time: 10 minutes

Cooking time: 20 minutes

Servings: 4 serving

Ingredients:

- Pepper to taste
- 3/4 cup onion, chopped
- 3/4 cup frozen corn kernels
- 3/4 teaspoon cumin
- 1 cup sweet potatoes, peeled and cut into 1/2-inch cubes
- 2 tablespoons flour
- 1/2 cup green bell pepper, seeded and chopped
- 1/2 cup dry white wine
- 14 ounces no-salt-added tomatoes
- 4 cups low-sodium chicken broth
- 1/2-pound cod, cut into bite-sized chunks
- 1/4 teaspoon red pepper flakes
- 1 and 1/2 teaspoons lime juice
- 1 clove garlic, minced
- Fresh parsley or cilantro for garnish (if desired)
- 3 slices low-sodium bacon, cut into pieces

Directions:

1. In a big saucepan, cook bacon until crisp over medium heat. Combine the onion, garlic, cumin, and pepper flakes in a mixing bowl. Cook for around 5 minutes, or until the onions are tender. Remove the pan from the fire and whisk in the flour. Cook for one minute and continually stirring.

2. Whisk in the chicken broth gradually. Add the onions, wine, peppers, and sweet potatoes and mix well. Bring to a boil, reduce to low heat, continue cooking for 10 minutes, or wait until the sweet potatoes are tender.

3. Toss in the fish and corn. Simmer for 2 to 3 minutes, or before the fish flakes easily when examined with a fork. Lime juice and pepper to taste. If needed, garnish with parsley or cilantro and serve in bowls.

19. Spicy Bean Soup

Preparation time: 10 minutes

Cooking time: 3 hours

Servings: 6 serving

Ingredients:

- 1 teaspoon black pepper
- 1 cup dried beans, assorted (navy, red, pinto, etc.)
- 1/4 teaspoon Tabasco sauce
- 1 cup diced carrot
- 6 ounces vegetable juice such as VB, spicy flavor
- 1/2 cup diced green bell pepper
- 3/4 cup diced celery
- 1 cup diced onion
- 1 cup diced ham
- 6 cups water

Directions:

1. In a big kettle, combine all of the ingredients. Allow for at least 3 hours of simmering time.

20.   Kidney Bean Stew

Preparation time: 10 minutes

Cooking time: 20 minutes

Servings: 4 serving

Ingredients:

- 1/2 teaspoon paprika
- 2 cups tomatoes, peeled and quartered
- 1 cup red bell pepper, seeded and chopped
- 1 cup celery, sliced
- 1 and 1/2 cup zucchini, sliced
- 8 ounces mushrooms, washed and sliced
- 3/4 cup carrot, sliced
- 1/2 cup dried kidney beans, soaked, cooked, and drained
- 1 and 1/2 cup onion, sliced
- Black pepper, fresh ground
- 1 tablespoon olive oil

Directions:

1. In a big saucepan, heat the oil and add the onion, red pepper, carrots, zucchini, and celery. Cook, wrapped, for 10 minutes before adding the mushrooms, onions, kidney beans, paprika, salt, and pepper to taste. Cook, wrapped, for an additional 10-15 minutes. Season to taste and serve.

CHAPTER 7: Non-Vegetarian Main Recipes

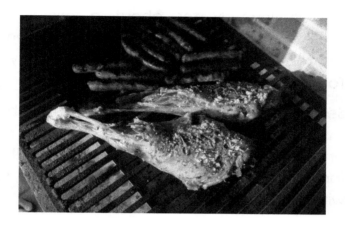

21. Pasta with Broccoli and Chicken

Preparation time: 10 minutes

Cooking time: 20 minutes

Servings: 4 serving

Ingredients:

- 3/4 cup low-sodium chicken broth
- 1/4 cup white wine
- 1 teaspoon dried basil
- 1 and 1/2 cups broccoli florets
- 2 garlic cloves, minced
- 1/2-pound bow tie pasta, cooked
- 1/2-pound boneless skinless chicken breasts, cut in l/2-inch strips

- 1/4 cup olive oil

Directions:

1. Heat the oil in a broad skillet over medium heat. Stir continuously for about a minute before sauteing the garlic. Cook until the chicken is fully cooked. Cook until the broccoli is crisp yet soft. Toss in the basil.

2. Season with pepper, wine, and chicken broth to taste. Cook for about 5 minutes. Toss the cooked and drained pasta into the skillet to mix it. Warm for 1–2 minutes. Serve the food. If required, sprinkle with grated Parmesan cheese.

22.   Chicken Alfredo

Preparation time: 10 minutes

Cooking time: 15 minutes

Servings: 4 serving

Ingredients:

- 4 ounces half-and-half
- 2 tablespoons grated Parmesan cheese
- 8 ounces no-salt-added tomato sauce
- 1 slice low-sodium bacon, cooked and crumbled
- 2 tablespoons dried basil
- 2 cloves garlic, minced
- 1 cup sliced mushrooms
- 1/2 cup chopped tomato
- 2 boneless chicken breasts, cut in chunks

Directions:

1. Cook the chicken in olive oil until it is golden brown. Cook on medium heat until the mushrooms begin to darken, then transform the chicken and add the onion, mushrooms, and garlic. Combine basil, pork, tomato sauce, and Parmesan cheese in a large mixing bowl.

2. Heat for 15 minutes on low. Remove the pan from the sun. Half-and-half can be added to the mixture. Mix well. Serve on top of spaghetti.

23.   Vidalia Onion Chicken Casserole

Preparation time: 10 minutes

Cooking time: 45 minutes

Servings: 6 serving

Ingredients:

- 1 tablespoon paprika
- 6 chicken breasts, boned and skinned
- 1 cup cooked rice
- 1 cup water
- 1/2 cup mayonnaise
- 2 large eggs, slightly beaten
- 1 cup grated Cheddar cheese
- 5 teaspoons olive oil, divided
- 1/2 cup sliced mushrooms
- 1/3 cup chopped Vidalia onions
- 10 ounces frozen broccoli

Directions:

1. Broccoli should be cooked according to package instructions. Drain the water and put it aside. 2 teaspoons olive oil, sautéed onions, and mushrooms until limp. Drain and toss with the broccoli. Remove from the equation. Combine the cheese, eggs, mayonnaise, water, and rice in a large mixing cup. Remove from the cup.

2. In the leftover olive oil, brown the chicken breasts. To make the casserole, combine the broccoli and cheese mixture in a greased, shallow baking tray. Sprinkle

3. paprika on top of the chicken breasts. Bake for 45 minutes at 350°F (180°C, gas mark 4) in an uncovered oven.

24. Quick Chicken and Mushroom Risotto

Preparation time: 10 minutes

Cooking time: 20 minutes

Servings: 4 serving

Ingredients:

- 1/2 cup frozen peas
- 1/8 teaspoon pepper
- 1 can cream of mushroom soup
- 14 and 1/2 ounces low-sodium chicken broth
- 1 cup long-grain rice, uncooked
- 1/2 cup carrot, sliced
- 1/2 cup onion, finely chopped
- 3/4-pound boneless skinless chicken breasts, cut into cubes
- 2 tablespoons unsalted butter, divided

Directions:

1. Cook chicken in 1 tablespoon melted butter in a 3-quart saucepan over medium-high heat until browned, stirring regularly. Remove the content and put it aside. Apply the leftover butter to the same saucepan.

2. Reduce heat to medium; cook onion, carrot, and rice, stirring continuously, until rice is browned. Combine the broth, soup, and pepper in a mixing bowl. Get to a simmer. Reduce the heat to a low

environment. Cook for 15 minutes, covered, stirring periodically.

3. Add the peas and the chicken that was set back. Cook, stirring regularly, for 5 minutes or until chicken is no longer yellow, rice is soft, and liquid has been absorbed.

25. Chicken Breasts Baked In Creamy Herb Sauce

Preparation time: 10 minutes

Cooking time: 35 minutes

Servings: 4 serving

Ingredients:

- 3 tablespoons lime juice
- 1/4 teaspoon thyme
- 1/4 teaspoon parsley
- 1/4 teaspoon coriander
- 1/4 teaspoon garlic powder
- 1/4 teaspoon celery seed
- 1/2 teaspoon oregano
- 1/2 teaspoon lime peel, grated
- 1/4 cup sour cream
- 1 cup plain yogurt
- 4 boneless skinless chicken breasts

Directions:

1. Preheat the oven to 375 degrees Fahrenheit (190 degrees Celsius, or gas mark 5). Place chicken breasts in a roasting pan coated with nonstick vegetable oil spray and set aside. Combine the other components in a mixing bowl. Bake for 20 minutes after brushing the chicken breasts with the mixture.

2. Remove the dish from the oven. Turn the chicken breasts over, baste with gravy, and bake for an additional 15 minutes or until the meat is tender.

3. Switch the oven off. Cover the chicken with foil and bake for 10 minutes. Remove the aluminum foil and place the chicken breasts on a serving dish with any leftover sauce.

26. Slow Cooker Chicken in Tomato Cream Sauce

Preparation time: 10 minutes

Cooking time: 1 hour 30 minutes

Servings: 6 serving

Ingredients:

- 1 and 1/2 cup mushrooms, sliced
- 1 cup frozen peas, thawed
- 8 ounces fettuccine
- 3/4 cup parmesan cheese, grated
- 2 egg yolks
- 1 cup fat-free evaporated milk
- 1 tablespoon basil
- 14- and 1/2-ounces canned tomatoes, drained and chopped
- 1 teaspoon garlic, minced
- 1/4 cup green onions, chopped
- 2 tablespoons olive oil
- 2 chicken breasts halves

Directions:

1. Brown chicken breasts in olive oil in a pan. In a slow cooker, position the chicken. Combine the green onions, garlic, peppers, and basil in a large mixing bowl. Cook on low for 7 to 9 hours,

covered. Remove the chicken from the pan and break it into bits.

2. Return the chicken to the oven. Combine the milk, egg yolks, and Parmesan cheese in a mixing cup. To thicken, cover, and cook on high for 30 minutes. Heat fettuccine according to box instructions as the sauce thickens; rinse. Combine the fettuccine, peas, and mushrooms in a large mixing bowl. Cook for 30 to 60 minutes on warm, covered.

27. Hawaiian Chicken

Preparation time: 10 minutes

Cooking time: 45 minutes

Servings: 4 serving

Ingredients:

- 1/2 cup coarsely chopped onion
- 1/2 cup chopped red bell pepper
- 4 chicken thighs
- 1/4 cup red wine vinegar
- 1/4 cup honey
- 8 ounces pineapple chunks

Directions:

1. Drain the pineapple and conserve the milk. Combine the juice, butter, and vinegar in a mixing bowl. In an 8 x 12-inch baking tray put the chicken. Overtop, strew pineapple, and tomatoes. Pour the juice mixture over the top. Bake for 45 minutes at 350°F (180°C, gas mark 4) or until chicken is cooked.

28.   Ranch Chicken Stir-Fry

Preparation time: 10 minutes

Cooking time: 10 minutes

Servings: 4 serving

Ingredients:

- 2 tablespoons water
- 16 ounces frozen winter vegetable mix, thawed
- 1 package ranch dressing mix
- 1/2-pound boneless skinless chicken breast, cut into strips
- 1 tablespoon olive oil

Directions:

1. In a big skillet, heat the vegetable oil. Toss in the chicken breast strips. To cover the chicken, whisk in the Ranch Salad Dressing Blend. Combine the thawed vegetable medley with the bath. 2 minutes of stir-frying

29.   Chicken Piccata

Preparation time: 10 minutes

Cooking time: 15 minutes

Servings: 4 serving

Ingredients:

- 1 tablespoon capers, drained, rinsed
- 2 tablespoons fresh lemon juice
- 1/4 cup vermouth
- 1/2 cup low-sodium chicken broth
- 1 teaspoon olive oil
- 2 tablespoons unsalted butter
- 1/2 teaspoon black pepper, freshly ground
- 4 boneless skinless chicken breasts

Directions:

1. Dry the chicken with a paper towel. Season with salt and pepper. In a heavy broad skillet, melt butter and oil over medium-high flame. Cook until the chicken is no longer pink, around 4 minutes per hand.

2. Remove from skillet and set aside to stay warm. Turn on the heat to heavy. In a skillet, combine the broth and vermouth. Cook until the liquid has been diminished by half, cleaning up any browned parts along the way.

3. Remove the pan from the flame.

4. Combine your lemon juice and capers in a mixing bowl. Place the chicken on plates and top with the sauce. If required, serve

5. the chicken with lemon slices as a garnish.

30. Chicken Marsala

Preparation time: 10 minutes

Cooking time: 15 minutes

Servings: 4 serving

Ingredients:

- 1/4 teaspoon pepper
- 1 teaspoon lemon juice
- 1/2 cup heavy cream
- 1/4 cup Marsala wine
- 1/2-pound mushrooms, thinly sliced
- 4 shallots, finely chopped
- 4 tablespoons butter, divided
- 4 boneless skinless chicken breasts

Directions:

1. Pound the breasts to a thickness of 1/4 inch with the flat (smooth) side of a meat mallet. 2 teaspoons butter, melted in a big frying pan over medium heat cook, rotating once, until chicken is lightly browned, around 2 minutes per hand. Remove the breasts and put them aside. In the same skillet, melt the remaining butter. Toss in the shallots and mushrooms. Cook for 3 to 5 minutes, or until mushrooms are finely browned.

2. Bring the Marsala to a simmer, cleaning off any browned pieces from the bottom of the pot. Return to a simmer with the cream and lemon

juice. To taste, season with pepper. Return the chicken to the pan

3. cook for 3 minutes, turning in the sauce to reheat and finish the cooking.

31. Chicken in Sour Cream Sauce

Preparation time: 10 minutes

Cooking time: 1 hour 10 minutes

Servings: 4 serving

Ingredients:

- 1/2 cup slivered almonds
- Pepper to taste
- 1 tablespoon green pepper, finely chopped
- 1/2 teaspoon thyme
- 2 tablespoons fresh parsley
- 1/2 teaspoon rosemary
- 1/2 cup sherry
- 1/2-pint fat-free sour cream
- 1/2 cup unsalted butter
- 2 pounds boneless skinless chicken breast

Directions:

In a pan, brown the chicken in butter. Placed in a casserole. Toss the chicken drippings with sour cream and sherry. Simmer for 10 minutes with the remaining ingredients. The mixture can be poured over chicken bits. Preheat oven to 350°F (180°C, or gas mark 4) and bake for 1 hour.

32.   French Chicken

Preparation time: 10 minutes

Cooking time: 15 minutes

Servings: 2 serving

Ingredients:

- 2 tablespoons heavy cream
- 3 tablespoons water
- 3 tablespoons vermouth
- 1 tablespoon mustard, coarse grain
- 1 tablespoon Dijon mustard
- 2 boneless skinless chicken breasts
- 1 tablespoon olive oil
- 1 tablespoon unsalted butter

Directions:

1. In a heavy-bottomed casserole, melt the sugar. Pour in the oil. Cook the chicken for around 2 or 3 minutes on either hand. Pour out some extra fat with care. Combine the mustards, vermouth, and water in a mixing bowl. Get the sauce to a low boil, cleaning off any brown bits from the pan's rim.

2. Cook for 10 minutes with the lid on. Check the chicken and see if it's cooked. Transfer the meat to individual serving dishes and keep warm. Mix in the milk thoroughly. Load the sauce over the chicken and eat.

33. Orange Burgundy Chicken

Preparation time: 10 minutes

Cooking time: 20 minutes

Servings: 4 serving

Ingredients:

- 4 boneless chicken breasts
- 1/4 cup burgundy wine
- 1/2 teaspoon cornstarch
- 1/4 cup orange marmalade

Directions:

1. Combine the first three components in a shallow saucepan. Cook, constantly stirring, until the sauce has thickened and is bubbling. On a charcoal or gas grill, cook chicken breasts until cooked, around 15 minutes. (Alternatively, it may be cooked in the oven.) Within the last 5 minutes of preparation, brush the sauce over the chicken. Serve the leftover sauce on top of the chicken.

34. Oriental Barbecued Pork Chops

Preparation time: 5 minutes

Cooking time: 3 hours

Servings: 4 serving

Ingredients:

- 1/2 cup no-salt-added tomato sauce
- 2 teaspoons sherry
- 1/2 teaspoon garlic powder
- 6 tablespoons Reduced-Sodium Soy Sauce
- 1/4 cup water
- 4 pork loin chops

Directions:

1. Get rid of the excess weight. Combine the soy sauce, ginger, sherry, and tomato sauce in a mixing cup. In a flat plate, pour over the beef.

2. Enable 3 hours in the refrigerator, sealed. Drain the marinade and place it in a small saucepan. Bring the water to a boil. Reduce heat to low and cook for 5 minutes. Grill until done, turning once over medium heat. Serve the beef with a fiery sauce.

35. Sweet and Sour Skillet Pork Chops

Preparation time: 5 minutes

Cooking time: 40 minutes

Servings: 6 serving

Ingredients:

- 1 cup celery, cut into strips
- 6 pineapple rings, juice packed
- 1/4 teaspoon cinnamon
- 1/4 tablespoon brown sugar substitute, such as Splenda 2 tablespoons cider vinegar
- Dash rosemary 1/2 cup pineapple juice
- 1 cup green bell pepper, cut into strips
- 6 pork chops

Directions:

1. Chops can be fully fat-free. In a skillet coated with nonstick vegetable oil mist, brown the meat on both sides. Chops can be eliminated. Combine pineapple juice, vinegar, and sugar substitute in a skillet. Combine the cinnamon and rosemary. Place the chops in the bath. Fill with celery.

2. Cook for 30 minutes at a low temperature. Green pepper strips can be included. On each chop, position a pineapple ring. Cook for another 10 minutes, covered. Place the chops on a serving platter and set aside. On top, arrange the pineapple and pepper strips. Pour the juice on top.

36.   Pineapple-Stuffed Pork Chops

Preparation time: 5 minutes

Cooking time: 15 minutes

Servings: 4 serving

Ingredients:

- 1 tablespoon chopped green onion
- 1/4 cup low-sodium ketchup
- 8 ounces pineapple slices
- 1/2 teaspoon dry mustard
- 4 pork loin chops, 1-inch thick

Directions:

1. To make way for the pineapple, cut a pocket in each chop. Drain the pineapple and save the juice. Two pineapple slices should be cut in half; the remaining pineapple should be torn up and put aside. Put a half pineapple slice in each chop's bag.

2. Preheat the grill to medium-high heat and barbecue for around 20 minutes, rotating once. Meanwhile, mix ketchup, green onion, mustard, and the stored pineapple juice and bits in a shallow saucepan. Bring to a boil, then reduce to low heat and cook for 10 minutes. 5 minutes more on the grill, brushing with sauce and spinning many times.

37. Memphis Spareribs

Preparation time: 5 minutes

Cooking time: 15 minutes **Servings:** 4 serving

Ingredients:

- 1/4 cup cider vinegar
- 2 pounds pork spareribs

Rub

- 1 teaspoon cayenne pepper
- 1 and 1/2 teaspoons black pepper
- 1/2 cup brown sugar

Sauce

- 1 teaspoon garlic powder
- 1/2 cup cider vinegar
- 1 teaspoon dry mustard
- 1 teaspoon onion powder
- 1/4 cup honey 1/2 teaspoon cayenne pepper
- 8 ounces no-salt-added tomato sauce

Directions:

1. Vinegar can be applied to the ribs. Combine the rub products and rub them onto the ribs. Cook until finished on the grill or in the smoker. Combine the sauce components as the ribs are frying. During the last 30 minutes of preparation, brush with sauce.

CHAPTER 8: Vegetarian Main Dishes

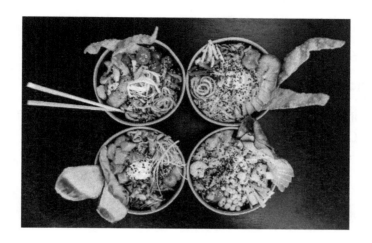

38.   Vegetable Soup

Preparation time: 10 minutes

Cooking time: 20 minutes

Servings: 8 servings

Ingredients:

- 2 cups shredded cabbage
- 1/2 cup sliced celery
- 1 teaspoon black pepper
- 2 turnips, peeled and diced
- 1 teaspoon basil
- 3 potatoes, peeled and diced
- 2 cups chopped tomato

- 3 carrots, peeled and sliced
- 1 teaspoon salt-free seasoning
- 12 ounces frozen mixed vegetables
- 1 onion, chopped
- 6 cups water

Directions:

1. In a big kettle, combine all of the ingredients. Cook until the vegetables are soft.

39. Beans and Barley

Preparation time: 10 minutes

Cooking time: 14 hours

Servings: 4 servings

Ingredients:

- 1/4 cup lentils, dried 1/4 cup pearl barley
- 1/2 cup split peas, dried 2 tablespoons fresh parsley, minced 1/2 teaspoon prepared mustard
- 4 cups low-sodium vegetable broth
- 1/2 cup mushrooms, chopped
- 1 cup carrot, chopped
- 3/4 cup onion, chopped
- 1 cup pinto beans, uncooked
- 1 cup white beans, uncooked

Directions:

1. White and pinto beans can be soaked overnight. 1 tablespoon vegetable reserve, sautéed onion, mushrooms, and carrots until soft. Add the drained beans, food reserve, mustard, and parsley to the sauteed vegetables. Get the water to a simmer.

2. Reduce the heat to a minimum, cover, and cook for 45 minutes. Combine the split peas, lentils, and barley in a large mixing dish. Place all of the ingredients in a broad slow cooker and cook on low for 12-14 hours.

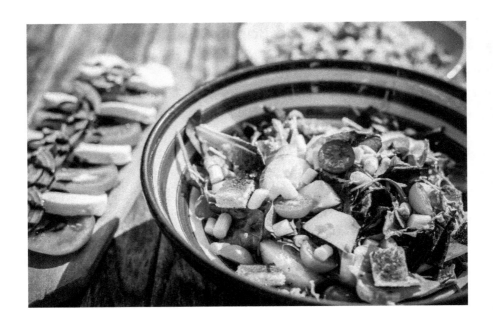

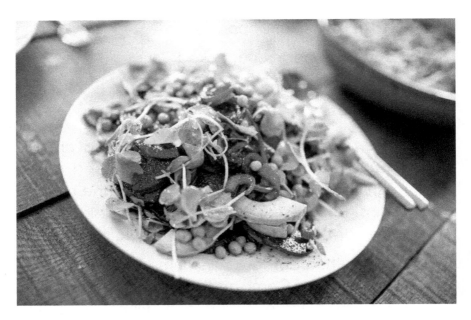

CHAPTER 9: Sauces, Dips & Dressing

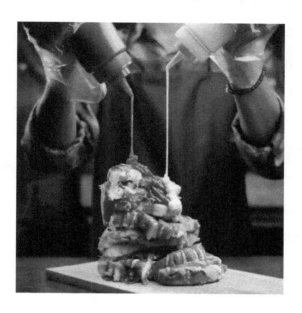

40.   Chili Sauce

Preparation time: 5 minutes

Cooking time: 1 and 1/2 hours

Servings: 48 servings

Ingredients:

- 1/2 cup cider vinegar
- 1 can no-salt-added tomato sauce
- 1/8 teaspoon basil
- 1/2 cup sugar
- 1/8 teaspoon cinnamon

- 1/2 cup chopped green pepper
- 1/4 teaspoon hot pepper sauce
- 1 tablespoon molasses
- 1 tablespoon brown sugar
- 1/8 teaspoon cloves
- 1 tablespoon lemon juice
- 1/8 teaspoon black pepper
- 1/2 cup chopped celery
- 1/8 teaspoon tarragon
- 1/2 cup chopped onion
- 1 can no-salt-added tomatoes

Directions:

1. In a big saucepan, add both of the ingredients. Bring to a boil, then reduce to low heat and continue to cook, uncovered, for 1 1/2 hours, or until the mixture has been reduced to half its original amount.

41. Reduced-Sodium Teriyaki Sauce

Preparation time: 5 minutes

Cooking time: 1 minute

Servings: 20 servings

Ingredients:

- Dash black pepper
- 2 slices ginger root
- 3 cloves garlic, crushed
- 1/2 cup sugar
- 2 tablespoons mirin wine
- 1 tablespoon sesame oil
- 1 cup Reduced-Sodium Soy Sauce

Directions:

1. In a saucepan, combine both ingredients and heat until sugar is dissolved. Refrigerate all leftovers.

42.   Reduced-Sodium Soy Sauce

Preparation time: 5 minutes

Cooking time: none

Servings: 48 servings

Ingredients:

- 1/4 cup reduced-sodium soy sauce
- 1/4 teaspoon garlic powder
- I/2 teaspoon ginger
- I/2 teaspoon black pepper
- 1/2 cups water, boiling
- 2 tablespoons molasses
- 4 tablespoons cider vinegar
- 4 tablespoons sodium-free beef bouillon

Directions:

1. Combine all of the ingredients mentioned above in a jar or an airtight container, shake to blend thoroughly. Cover and seal tightly. This may be stored in the fridge indefinitely.

CHAPTER 10: Slow Cooker Favorite

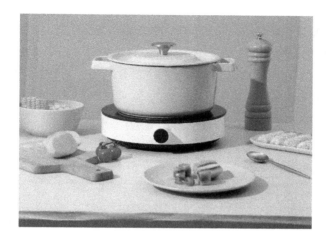

43. Lemon Roast Chicken

Preparation time: 10 minutes

Cooking time: 7 hours 10 minutes

Servings: 1 serving

Ingredients:

- Rosemary
- 1 tbsp. Lemon juice
- 1/4 cup water
- 1 tbsp. coconut oil
- 1 clove minced garlic
- 1 tsp. Oregano
- 1 dash Pepper
- 1 dash Salt

- 2 pieces skinless chicken

Directions:

1. Chicken can be washed and seasoned with salt and pepper. Fill the cavity of the chicken with part of the oregano and garlic. In a frying pan, boil the coconut oil.

2. Brown the chicken on both sides before placing it in the crockpot. Garlic and oregano can be sprinkled on top. Stir in a little water to loosen the brown bits in the pan.

3. Cover and pour into a crockpot. Cook for 7 hours on low. When the cooking is over, squeeze in the lemon juice. Place the chicken on a cutting board and carve it. Remove all excess fat. Fill a sauce bowl halfway with juice. Serve with rosemary and a squeeze of lemon juice on top of the chicken.

CHAPTER 11: Side Dishes

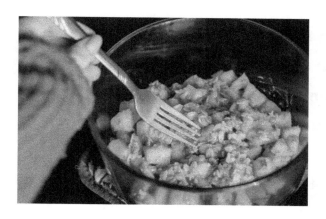

44.   Balsamic Onions

Preparation time: 10 minutes

Cooking time: 1 hour

Servings: 4 serving

Ingredients:

- 1/4 cup alsamic vinegar
- 4 medium onions
- 1 tablespoon olive oil

Directions:

1. Turnips can be steamed for 15 minutes over boiling water before fork tender. Drain turnips and combine with garlic and butter in a food processor or blender. Blend until smooth, incorporating more skim milk if necessary.

45. Fruit and Vegetable Curry

Preparation time: 10 minutes

Cooking time: 1 hour

Servings: 6 serving

Ingredients:

- 1 and 1/2 cups water
- 2 tablespoons olive oil
- 1/4 teaspoon ground cloves
- 1 teaspoon ginger root, minced
- 1/2 teaspoon fennel seeds
- 1 and 1/2 tablespoons coriander
- 1/2 teaspoon cayenne
- 1 teaspoon turmeric
- 1 and 1/2 teaspoons cinnamon
- 1/4 teaspoon cardamom
- 1 and 1/2 tablespoons cumin
- 3 cups zucchini, quartered and sliced
- 2 cloves garlic, minced
- 1 cup fresh green beans
- 4 cups onion, coarsely chopped
- 2 tablespoons fresh lemon juice
- 2 apples, cored and cubed
- 1/2 cup raisins

- 1 cup dried apricots, chopped
- 1/2 cup red bell pepper, diced

Directions:

1. Preheat the oven to 375 degrees Fahrenheit (190 degrees Celsius, gas mark 5). Using vegetable oil paint, lightly coat a shallow roasting plate.

2. Remove some loose skins from the onions and wash them. Olive oil can be applied to the onions.

3. Bake for 45 minutes to 1 hour, or until the potatoes are soft. Break onions in half and drizzle with balsamic vinegar. Serve immediately.

46. Easy Curried Vegetables

Preparation time: 10 minutes

Cooking time: 10 minutes

Servings: 4 serving

Ingredients:

- 1/2 cup coarsely chopped onion
- 2 cups sliced zucchini
- 1 tablespoon curry powder
- 2 cups no-salt-added canned tomatoes

Directions:

1. For 10 minutes, sauté the onions in the fat. Continue to sauté, stirring continuously, for 3 minutes after introducing the garlic, ginger, and spices. Stir in the zucchini and water to prevent the spices from sticking to the jar. Cook for 10 minutes with the lid on. Combine the green beans, apples, peppers, and dried apricots in a large mixing bowl.

2. Cook for around 30 minutes, sealed, on low heat. To stop sticking, stir regularly and add a little more water if necessary. Stir in the raisins and lemon juice until the fruit and vegetables are soft.

47. Curried Vegetables

Preparation time: 10 minutes

Cooking time: 10 minutes

Servings: 4 serving

Ingredients:

- 1/4 teaspoon garlic powder
- 1/2 cup coarsely chopped onion
- 1/2 cup coarsely chopped green bell peppers
- 1 cup cubed zucchini
- 1 tablespoon curry powder
- 3 cups no-salt-added canned tomatoes

Directions:

1. In a saucepan, combine all of the ingredients. Cook, sometimes stirring, until the onion and zucchini are soft.

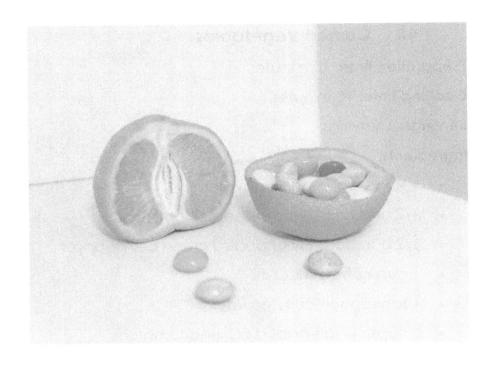

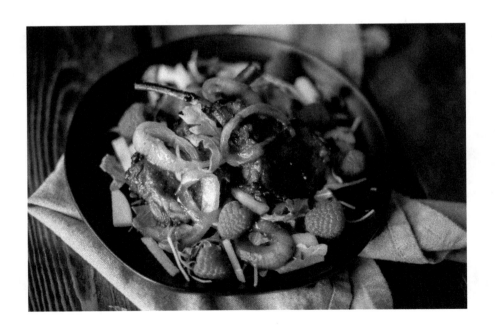

CHAPTER 12: Fish & Seafood Recipes

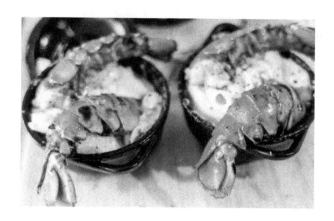

48. Garlic Scallops

Preparation time: 10 minutes

Cooking time: 10 minutes

Servings: 4 servings

Ingredients:

- 2 tablespoons lemon juice
- 2 tablespoons dried parsley flakes
- 3 cloves garlic, minced
- 2 tablespoons unsalted butter 1-pound scallops
- Pepper to taste 3 tablespoons flour

Directions:

1. Combine flour and pepper in a small dish. Toss in the scallops to coat. In a pan, melt the fat. Cook,

stirring regularly, for two minutes after adding the garlic.

2. Cook, turning periodically until scallops are cooked through, around 5 minutes. Add parsley and lemon juice to conclude.

49. Fluffy Shrimp Omelet

Preparation time: 10 minutes

Cooking time: 15 minutes

Servings: 4 servings

Ingredients:

- Pepper to taste 1/2 cup Swiss cheese, grated
- 1/2 cup mushrooms
- 3 tablespoons unsalted butter, divided
- 6 eggs, separated
- 8 ounces shrimp, cooked

Directions:

1. Preheat the oven to 350 degrees Fahrenheit (180 degrees Celsius, or gas mark 4) 2 teaspoons, sugar, sautéed mushrooms and green onions. Egg whites should be rigid. Egg yolks and pepper can be whisked together in a separate dish. Fold the beaten egg whites into the mixture. Then substitute the seafood, mushrooms, onions, and grated cheese. Gently fold the bits together.

2. In a strong, ovenproof pan, melt the remaining 1 tablespoon fat. Spread the omelet mixture equally in the pan. Brown the bottom of the pan for 3-5 minutes over low heat. Then bake for 5-10 minutes at 350°F (180°C, or gas mark 4) until a knife inserted in the middle comes out clean.

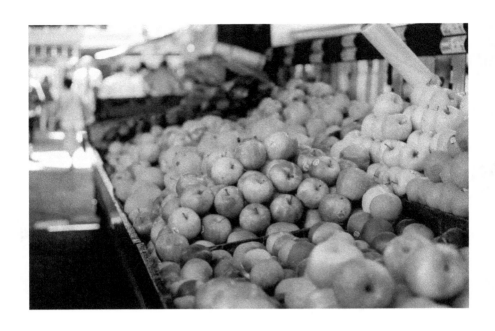

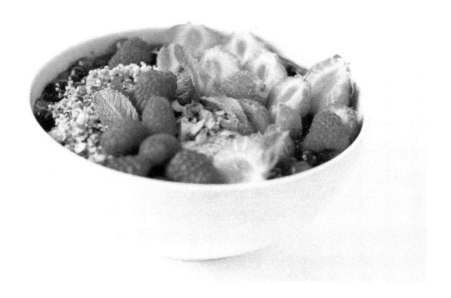

CHAPTER 13: Recipes for Holiday

50. The Big Veggie Stir-Fry

Preparation time: 5 minutes

Cooking time: 10 minutes

Servings: 4 serving

Ingredients:

- 4 scallions, chopped
- 2 cloves garlic, minced
- 2 stems lemongrass, thinly sliced
- ¼ teaspoon hot pepper flakes
- 1 red bell pepper, chopped
- 2 tablespoons rice vinegar
- 2 cups chopped bok choy
- 1½ cups water
- 5 cups broccoli florets
- 1 tofu, cut into 1-inch cubes
- 1 zucchini, chopped
- 2 teaspoons reduced-sodium soy sauce
- 4 cups shredded cabbage
- ¼ cup pineapple juice
- 2 teaspoons cornstarch
- 2 tablespoons tahini

- 2 tablespoons sesame seeds
- 1 tablespoon minced fresh ginger

Directions:

1. Combine the ginger, garlic, tahini, hot pepper flakes, pineapple juice, rice vinegar, soy sauce, and 14 cups of water in a shallow mixing dish. Remove from the dish.

2. Stir-fry tofu for 5 minutes over high heat, or until slightly browned, in a big wok rubbed with oil. Transfer to a bowl and cover with plastic wrap to stay wet.

3. Broccoli, bok choy, zucchini, red pepper, cabbage, and lemongrass, as well as 34–1 cup of water, go into the wok. Cook, covered, over medium-high heat until crisp yet soft, around 15 minutes (about 10 minutes).

4. In a wok, combine the tofu and the veggie mixture, then apply the sauce mixture. Stir-fry until fully hot (about 2 minutes).

5. Combine cornstarch and 3 tablespoons water in a small bowl and stir into wok. Cook for 2–3 minutes, or until the sauce has thickened. To change the quality, more water may be applied. Add scallions and sesame seeds to the end. Serve with Lentils and Herbed Barley.

6. Tofu may be substituted with 1 chicken breast, sliced into slices, shrimp, or scallops if needed.

Conclusion

We hope that this book marks the start of the road to long-term wellbeing and lively life. Many of the tips might be different from something you've done previously, and we recognize that you and others around you may need to make drastic lifestyle changes. It isn't often easy to alter, but it can be highly satisfying. It would be a wonderful feeling to see your diabetes reversing and maybe vanish, particularly knowing that you provided the chance by giving your body the nutrients it requires to do its job.

CPSIA information can be obtained
at www.ICGtesting.com
Printed in the USA
BVHW041439250621
610376BV00009B/1889